I0412070

Herbal Antibiotics For Beginners:

Natural Home Remedies to Cure Yourself, Prevent Illnesses and Infections

By

Sherri Neal

ISBN-13: 978-1507845837

Table of Contents

Herbal Antibiotics For Beginners: Natural Home Remedies to Cure Yourself, Prevent Illnesses and Infections

By Sherri Neal

© Copyright 2015 Sherri Neal

Reproduction or translation of any part of this work beyond that permitted by section 107 or 108 of the 1976 United States Copyright Act without permission of the copyright owner is unlawful. Requests for permission or further information should be addressed to the author.

This publication is designed to provide accurate and authoritative information in regard to the subject matter covered. This work is sold with the understanding that the publisher is not engaged in rendering legal, accounting, or other professional services. If legal advice or other expert assistance is required, the services of a competent professional person should be sought.

First Published, 2015

Printed in the United States of America

Introduction

Herbal antibiotics have been used for centuries to ward off diseases and viral infections. These herbs are free of side effects, inexpensive and easily accessible, in fact, most of them is already found in your kitchen. All these qualities make natural antibiotics a great alternate for synthetic antibiotics.

Researches suggest that pharmaceutical antibiotics contain toxins and synthetic chemicals and can produce side effects of varying nature. Side effects may include gastrointestinal problems, allergic reactions, kidney infections and inefficient immune function. More importantly, synthetic antibiotics become redundant as the time goes by and cause to the spread and growth of antibiotic resistant bacteria, meaning antibiotic will stop working against a disease or infection and will not support in healing a wound. One of the dangerous bacteria is MRSA which is the acronym for "methicillin-resistant Staphylococcus aureus" and can resist against most of the antibiotics.

Chapter 1. What Are The Harmful Effects of Pharmaceutical Antibiotics?

Pharmaceutical antibiotics are lifesavers indeed. They are used to treat a number of infections and diseases and help save many of lives each day. However many harmful effects are also associated with them.

One of the major issues is side effects and reactions which are commonly observed after taking antibiotics. The side effects can be range anywhere from mild to severe in intensity. Feeling nausea, upset stomach and diarrhea are very common side effects. Some people may caught allergic reactions and very few of them, may end up dying from it but it happens very rarely.

The function of an antibiotic is killing bacteria but a synthetic antibiotic cannot differentiate between good and bad bacteria and keeps on killing both types of bacteria. Eventually, a person might be cured from the certain disease but it will leave a harmful effect on immune system and will increase the chances of the attack of some other disease.

Pharmaceutical antibiotics are prescribed by doctors and medical professionals. Once the course is started, you are bound to complete it. If you stop taking the medicine in the middle, your disease will get worse; bacteria may change its form and grew stronger. You will have to start it all over again and have to take a much higher dose to get rid of the disease.

Antibiotics cannot be used without the consultation and recommendation of any professional and their unnecessary and excessive use can have a damaging effect on your body and overall health.

Many factors are considered before prescribing an antibiotic such as any allergic reaction in the past with any antibiotic or any other medicine patient is taking because interaction with other medicine may lead to some kind of allergic reaction.

Chapter 2. Why Herbal Antibiotics Are Great Alternative for Artificial Antibiotics?

The overall effectiveness of herbal antibiotics makes them an ideal replacement of artificial antibiotics and this statement is also backed by many scientific researches.

Firstly, herbal antibiotics do not possess toxins and harmful, synthetic chemicals. They are safe for everyone and can be taken anytime and in any age to eliminate bacteria causing infections.

Herbal antibiotics have virtually no side effects no matter in which quantity they are taken because they are natural and pure and are devoid of chemicals. They are easy to ingest and adapt.

The regular intake of herbal antibiotics naturally boosts immune system and helps you defend from various infectious bacteria. If they are taken during a condition, they will cleanse the blood and help eliminate the bacteria.

Natural antibiotics can be taken without the consultation of your medical doctor but you have to be very sure on what kind of herb or food will help you fight against a certain disease because not every herbal antibiotic is useful against every type of disease.

The infectious diseases that can be cured with herbal antibiotics

A number of viral and bacterial infections can be treated with herbal antibiotics but if infection is of severe nature and is getting out of control, it is advisable to rush to the doctor for proper medical treatment.

Herbal antibiotics are quite useful against mild viral infections such as cold, flu, cough, sneeze and earaches and positive effects are quite visible when natural herbs are used to cure from these infections.

Many intestinal problems such as vomiting, upset stomach and painful bowel movements or constipation can be successfully treated with herbs and foods available in your kitchen or grown in your garden.

The intake of herbal antibiotics in severe health conditions such as herpes, hepatitis, dengue, diarrhea and pneumonia can also help fight against bacteria or can be used to support or complement the medical treatment.

Chapter 3. Common Herbal Antibiotics

A number of herbs, scrubs and foods contain antibacterial properties and are used as a home remedy for multiple infectious diseases. It means herbs not only enhance the taste of your meals but also prevents you from various diseases. The following are some of the herbs that are most commonly used as antibiotics.

Ginger

Ginger root is mostly known for culinary use and is an important ingredient of Asian cooking but it is also used as a home remedy to treat multiple health conditions. It is considered quite effective against nausea and relieves from uneasiness or stomach queasiness experienced before the vomiting. Ginger helps calm down the stomach and also aids in reducing the problems accompanied with it such as gas trouble, bloating and indigestion. If kids are having worms in their intestine, the intake of ginger will help remove worms from the stomach especially the roundworms.

Ginger also helps improve the blood circulation and reduces the risk of blood clotting and eventually the heart problems. The patients of migraine can also use ginger to reduce headaches, dizziness and vertigo. Ginger is believed to be useful against chronic disease arthritis as well. The patients of arthritis suffer from immobility, extreme pain and stiffness. If they take three to four grams of ginger powder daily, it will help reduce the visible symptoms of arthritis.

Ginger is considered most effective when it is taken in the form of either powder or essential oil. But like any other thing, the excessive ingestion of ginger can be harmful and cause a lot of sweating and fluids out of your skin.

Garlic

In many parts of the world, cooking is considered incomplete without using garlic. Many add this ingredient to get a pungent flavor in their dish while many other use it to have a strong aroma coming out of their cooking pot.

As an antibiotic, garlic seems to have limitless effectiveness. It can be used to combat multiple diseases ranging from common flu to chronic fungal infections to cancer and garlic's organic pesticide properties make it a popular herbal remedy. If someone has a tendency of cold, cough or flu in winters, eating garlic as soon as the slightest of the hint is received will help prevent from these viral infections and will also soothe the bronchus, a passage that takes air into the lungs. If it is difficult to eat a raw garlic, garlic based soup can be made to get similar kind of benefits.

Garlic is a great anti infective natural drug whether it is taken through the mouth or applied directly on to the skin to cure may infections such as athlete's foot. Garlic contains a compound known as ajoene which is quite effective against the fungus causing athlete's foot. Garlic whether it is eaten fresh or in the form of dried extract is a successful treatment for vaginal yeast infection. Many researches also suggest that regular use of garlic may lower the risk of many types of cancers such as breast, bladder, skin, and stomach cancers.

Garlic is also considered good for the health of the heart. It prevents blood from clotting, improves it flow to the heart and throughout the body, thereby reduces the risk of heart attack.

Turmeric

Turmeric is a cooking ingredient found in every kitchen cabinet. The herb is not mostly used fresh. Its leaves are dried and grinned into a orange colored powder. It adds a very sharp taste and aroma in the meals.

Besides culinary purposes, it has a very long history of curative use. Turmeric contains antiviral, antibacterial and anti inflammatory properties, making it a natural treatment for multiple infections and viral diseases. A substance named lipopolysaccharide is commonly found in turmeric which helps boost immune system and prevents from seasonal viruses such as flu, cold and coughs. Turmeric has a magical effect on cuts and wounds. Rubbing turmeric on open wound not only help clean it from bacteria but also speeds up the healing process and naturally repairs the skin damaged with the cut, wound or burn.

Turmeric is a very important part of Asian culture. Many countries of the region use it as a natural healing agent. Traditionally, a spoon of turmeric powder is mixed in the warm milk. Taking this milk can heal up the internal wounds, make bones strong and work as a body detox. Scientific researches reveal some more benefits of turmeric. According to cancer research UK, turmeric can destroy cancer cells and prevent them from growing and spreading. Another study suggested that chemotherapy, a treatment for cancer combined with turmeric killed more cancer cells than the chemotherapy alone.

Thyme

Thyme is an herb widely used throughout the history for bringing flavor and delightful smell in the dishes but its benefits as an herbal medicine also worth mentioning. Thyme relieves from cold, cough, bronchitis emphysema and asthma especially the tea made with this is quite helpful in fight against these seasonal viruses. You can also add mind leaves to enhance the flavor and to get a refreshing feel. Gargling with thyme mixed warm water is also effective for sore throat and relaxes the airway passage of bronchus.

Thyme is common home remedy to treat various eye related problems such as watery eyes, burning eyes and temporary blur vision. It can also successfully deal with other viral infections that arise during the winter and spring season like symptoms of fever, headache, fatigue and running nose. If parasites are found in the digestive tract, taking thyme tea will help eliminate them naturally. The intestinal parasites that can be successfully eliminated with this herb are hookworms, tapeworms, pinworms and roundworms. Combining thyme with other herbs such as rosemary and chamomile will produce even greater results. The procedure is simple. Put thyme and other herbs in a paper bag. Do not forget to make holes in the bag to ensure the circulation of air and place it in a high temperature room for few weeks. If you are in a bit hurry and cannot wait for that long, dry these herbs in microwave. Once dried, make an infusion of the herbs. Also add a piece of ginger root and drink this infusion or tea thrice a day regularly until worms are gone from the digestive tract.

Chamomile

Chamomile is a great combatant against stomach related problems and comforts excessive gas and bloating, upset stomach, cramps, stomach flu and bowel pain. The herb is an excellent choice for all those who complaints about menstrual cramps, pain and improper sleep due to premenstrual syndrome.

If you have kids in the house, this herb is a must for your kitchen cabinet. It helps calm uneasiness and restlessness in children and its light taste and smell also make it tolerable for the children. Otherwise, a medicine with a strong smell and flavor is not easy to swallow and digest. Chamomile makes both adults and children calm and help them fall asleep. It is proven treatment of insomnia as well.

If you are prone to seasonal allergic reactions, use chamomile regularly during the season or even before it starts as a precautionary measure. It will prevent from intensifying allergic reactions and at least reduce it to a great extent. For adults, cup of chamomile tea two to three times a day is very helpful. It will also ease your mind and relieves from fatigue thoughts but it will not create hindrance in driving and other tasks which require full concentration. For children, who cannot take tea regularly; make a cream out of chamomile herb. Rubbing this herbal cream all over diaphragm, the area across the rib cage, will soothe and relaxes the stiff muscles and will make breathing easier.

Basil

Basil leaves are widely used for seasoning in cooking but this herb is a also an answer to lots of health issues. Basil contains various essential nutrients that help restore or maintain overall health. Chewing the leaves of basil reduces seasonal flu, fever and common cold and also helps bring down the high temperature to a normal temperature.

The basil leaves also decreases the risk of malaria and dengue fever. The consumption of basil leaves help cure from dengue fever and you can also use it as a complementary treatment to make the conventional medical treatment more effective and result oriented. The tree of basil is a natural mosquito repellent. If basil is grown inside the house, its smell will keep mosquitoes away. Mosquito is the source of the dengue fever and keeping it away from you and your house means that you will no longer become a prey to this seasonal fever. You can also rub the basil essential oil across you body to prevent yourself from mosquito sting.

If you want to get rid of bad breath, make a powder with dried basil leaves and mix it with mustard oil. Apply it on your teeth and gums and rub gently with your fingers. It is a great replacement of conventional toothpastes and will not only prevent you from bad breath but also improves the overall oral health.

Peppermint

The mint family comprises of many types of mint plants but peppermint is probably the most popular of them all. Due to its refreshing, cooling effect, peppermint is frequently used as a main ingredient of herbal medicine and skincare products.

Peppermint is a well known natural treatment for stomach problems. There are many types of teas available in the market for upset stomach but their strong and unpleasant odor makes them difficult to drink. On the other hand, the tea made with peppermint leaves is a refreshing way to deal with nausea, stomach pain, irritable bowel and intestinal cramps. Peppermint is equally suitable and effective for infants as well. If any infant is suffering from stomach problem, give him a teaspoon of peppermint tea. If he is unable to take it through mouth, soak a cloth in the peppermint tea and rub this cloth gently on the infant's belly. The gentle rubbing will relieve the child from stomach cramp and pain.

Peppermint contains an organic compound called menthol which is known for its antiseptic, antiviral and antifungal properties and cooling effect. It will relieve from itching, burning and insect bites but the affect will be temporary and the patient will require proper medication in order to fully recover from these problems.

Clove

Clove is floral bud with a strong smell and flavor. Aside from culinary use, it is used as an herbal remedy for various diseases in many countries across the globe. Clove, especially the oil obtained from the bud, is quite effective against tooth related problems such as toothache and tooth decay. You might also have observed that clove oil is often found in toothpastes that claim to relieve from tooth problems.

The presence of antibacterial properties makes clove a great natural treatment for wounds, cuts, bruises, insect bites and viral infections such as cholera, malaria and scabies. It can also work well for common viral infections like cough, flu and sore throat. Simply chewing on the few cloves can soothe the throat and makes the passage free of the pain experienced during the sore throat. Gargling with clove oil is a even better choice for getting rid of sore throat.

If you are having insomnia and restless nights, mix few drops of clove oil with any carrier oil, pour the oil on your forehead and massage it gently. It will also remove anxiety, stress, mental exhaustion and headaches and help fall into a deep and satisfying sleep.

Chapter 4. Natural Herbal Remedies

These are the few recipes of making natural herbal medicine at home. The ingredients will likely be found in your kitchen cabinet in the form of spices or as a seasoning ingredient. If not, they can be easily purchased from grocery store near to your home. These herbal remedies are useful to ward off various diseases, infections and viruses.

Home remedies for common cold and flu

Boil water in a large bowl and add 5 to 10 drops of thyme oil or eucalyptus oil depending on your preference. Now grab a towel and cover both the bowl and your head in such way that it will lock steam inside. Take a deep breathe through your nose and continue the procedure for further five to ten minutes but do not lower your face too much into the steam because it can damage your skins and eyes. This herbal remedy will make you breathe easy and will help reduce cold and flu.

Grab a clove of garlic and place it inside your mouth. Take deep breathes so the fumes can reach to the throat and in to the lungs or you can just chew a piece of garlic and drink water to swallow it.

Add a small ½ piece of ginger, 2 cinnamon sticks into six cups of water and bring the mixture to the boil. Once boiled, take the tea off the heat and add a teaspoon of honey and stir. Drink the tea while warm and reap its benefits.

Home remedies for diarrhea

The disease of diarrhea is characterized with abdominal cramps, loose stools, excessive bowel movements, sickness and vomiting and these symptoms also suggest that digestive system is not working properly. There can be a number of reasons causing diarrhea such as ingesting poison, growth of a certain kind of bacteria, deficiency of fiber or an enzyme, intestinal parasites and allergic reaction of a food.

Chamomile tea is great way to treat diarrhea and symptoms associated with it. To make this tea, add one teaspoon of chamomile flowers with the same quantity of peppermint leaves in a pot full of water and boil it for 5 to 10 minutes. Then, strain out the herbs and drink this tea at least thrice a day. The tea can also help boost digestive system.

Ginger is also a great tonic for digestive problems. Blend a small piece of ginger with one teaspoon of honey and ingest this mixture to stimulate digestive system and to ensure stomach health.

Home remedies for cough

Coughing is an annoying thing indeed especially continues cough can put a person into a constant state of restlessness. The following are few herbal remedies to ease off coughing.

Thyme is an herb which relaxes the respiratory tract and helps reduce coughing. Grab some fresh thyme or you can also use one tablespoon of dried thyme and add it to the boiling water. Let it steep for a while. Then, take the herb out of the mixture and take sips of the tea. You can also add a teaspoon of honey to enhance the flavor and to get better results.

The infusion of basil and cloves can also help reduce coughing. In a pot, add five to eight basil leaves, few cloves, cup of water and a pinch of salt to add taste. Put the mixture on the stove and heat up until boil properly. It will approximately take eight to ten minutes to bring the boil. Pour the mixture through a strainer into a cup and drink it to ease off coughing. You can also gargle with basil based warm water to get desired results.

Home remedies for sore throat

Sore throat is the pain and irritation of the throat which is caused by any viral or bacterial infection. The common symptoms include dry and itchy throat, swelling in throat, muffled voice and difficulty in swallowing and sipping. Few of the home remedies to deal with sore throat are:

Add few drops of eucalyptus oil in boiling water and pour this water into a large bowl. Then lean forward to inhale the steam coming out of the bowl. Drape the towel around your head and bowl and trap the steam inside. Keep on taking the steam through your nose but avoid being too close to the bowl as it may cause harm to your skin. This simple remedy will prove soothing for the pain of the throat and will also help ease congested breathe.

You can also make a herbal syrup at your home to relieve sore throat. All you need is few cloves and a cup of honey. Mix both the ingredients together and refrigerate them overnight. Take the mixture out of the refrigerator in the morning, remove the cloves from it and take a spoonful of honey. Clove will help reduce the pain while honey will soothe the burning throat.

Home remedies for hepatitis

Hepatitis refers to the inflammation of liver. It generally occurs with the overdose of a drug, consumption of excessive alcohol or as a result of a viral infection. Hepatitis can be of various types such as A, B, C so it is necessary to have blood test before taking medicine. You can reduce the disease with home remedies as well.

Green tea is known for its liver protective properties. It contains a powerful antioxidant called catechin which is believed to do repair work with the cells damaged because of toxins. If herbal tea is taken three times a day on regular basis, it will prove a great treatment for hepatitis but it is advisable to take it as a complementary treatment or a treatment that can support your conventional medical treatment.

Turmeric is also considered a combatant against hepatitis C. It contains antioxidant and anti inflammatory properties that can improve the functioning of liver and protect damaged cells. You can take 1 teaspoon of turmeric in the powder form to observe its effects on hepatitis.

Home remedies for better sleep

Insufficient or broken sleep directly affects your work and productivity. If the problem continues, it might convert into a disorder known as insomnia. In order to get a proper deep sleep, you can use many herbal remedies such as:

Lemon balm, a member of mint family has a long history for promoting sleep, relieving from anxiety and depression and easing off pain and restlessness. It can be taken either in the form of tea or as a supplement to get a better and proper sleep.

Chamomile also has a calming and soothing effect on your mind which eventually aids in deep and sufficient sleep. Researches also suggest that chamomile does not have a direct effect on the sleep instead it reduces the anxiety disorder and relaxes the nerves.

Home remedies for healing wounds

Generally, conventional medicines are preferred for healing wounds, cuts and bruises. But few organic remedies can also be used to successfully treat wounds and scrapes.

Aloe vera is mostly known as burn relief hub but it can also treat scrapes, wounds and cuts. This herbaceous plant contains a gel which is often found in many skincare products as well. Applying this gel directly on the affected area provides instant relieve from pain and also speeds up the healing process.

Honey is another natural treatment for healing wounds and speeding up the recovery. The dressing of honey instantly heals wounds and scrapes and prevents from infection as well. Manuka honey, produced in New Zealand and Australia, is found quite effective in this regard.

Home remedies for boosting immune system

If you have strong immune system, it will naturally defend you from many diseases. There are several home remedies that can help boost your immune system and indirectly prevent you from various infections and diseases.

Garlic is credited with having such ingredients that can boost your immune system. Make a regular part of your cooking or add cloves of garlic right before serving the food to get its benefits. If you are daring enough, you can even chew it to stimulate your immune system.

Conclusion

Herbal antibiotics are a natural way to treat diseases and infections. They herbal remedies are popular today not because they were used by our forefathers but because they are actually effective and useful and their effectiveness is backed by many scientific researches as well.

Thank You Page

I want to personally thank you for reading my book. I hope you found information in this book useful and I would be very grateful if you could leave your honest review about this book. I certainly want to thank you in advance for doing this.

If you have the time, you can check my other books too.

www.ingramcontent.com/pod-product-compliance
Lightning Source LLC
Chambersburg PA
CBHW070527290526
45790CB00003B/1334